Large Print

Mandala Coloring Book

For Visual Impaired Adults & Teenagers

Bold Lines, High Contrast, Large Patterns

Rachel Mintz

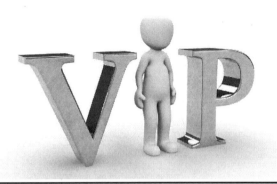

Join Our Coloring Books VIP Group
Members Get Giveaways, Deep Discount Offers,
Win Prizes – Visit Site To Join (It's Free)

www.ColoringBookHome.com

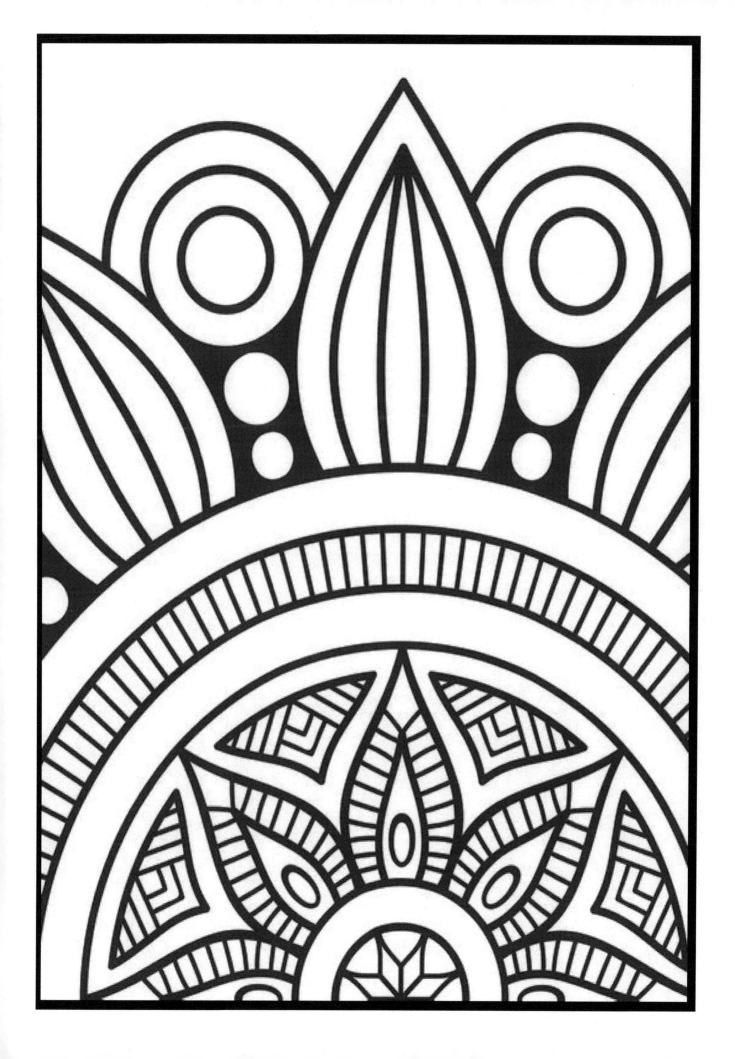

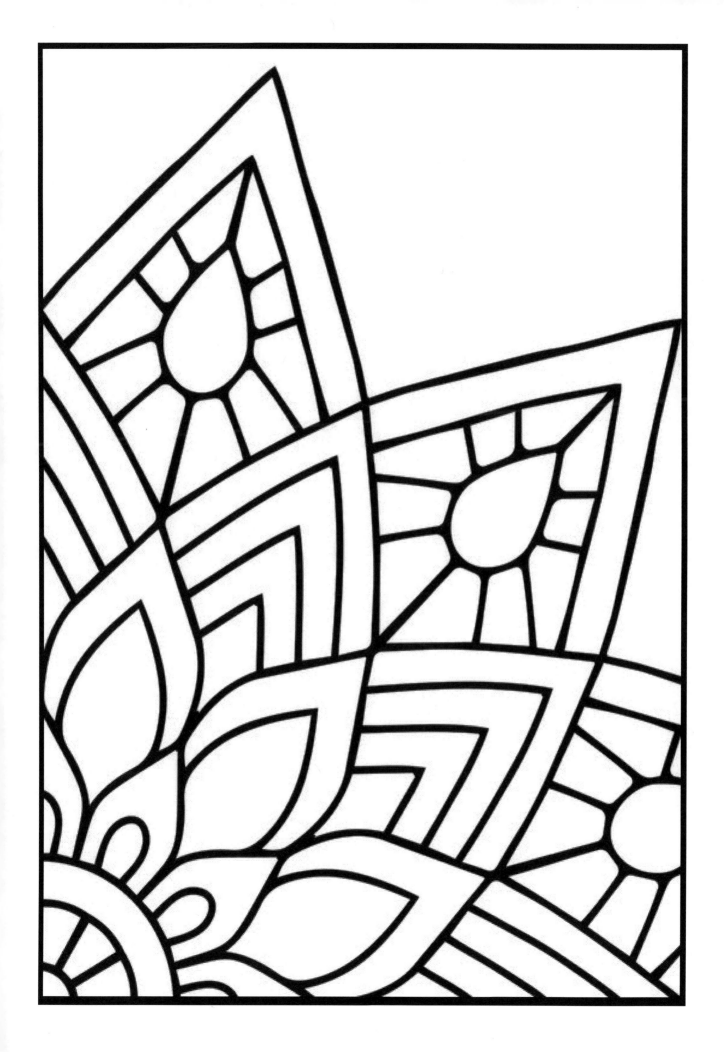

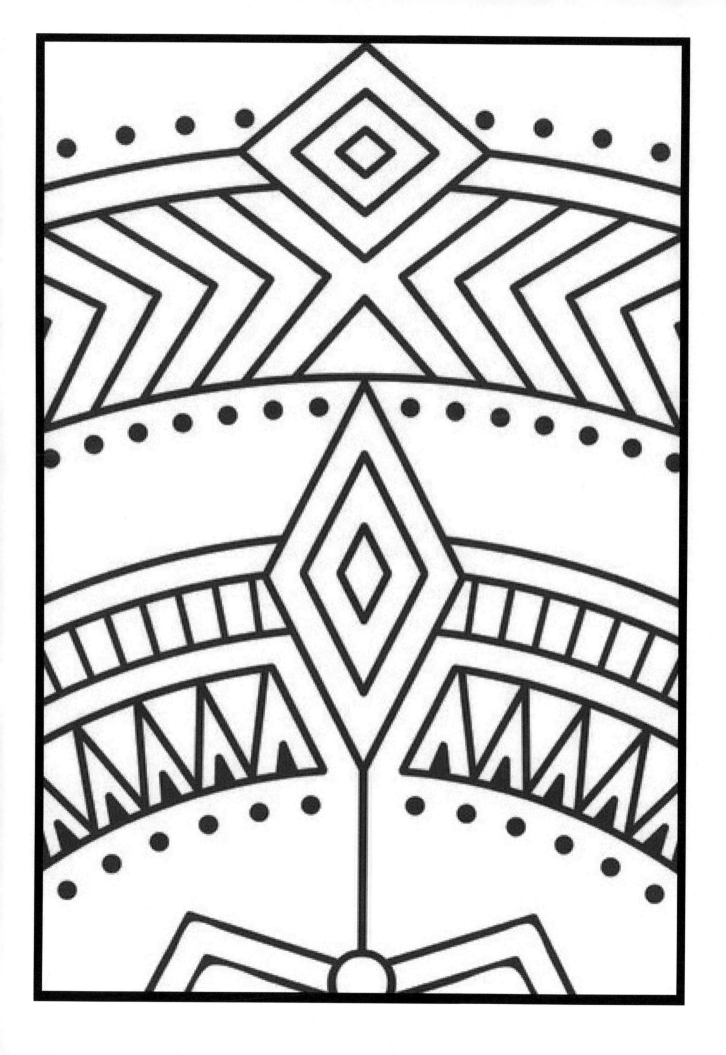

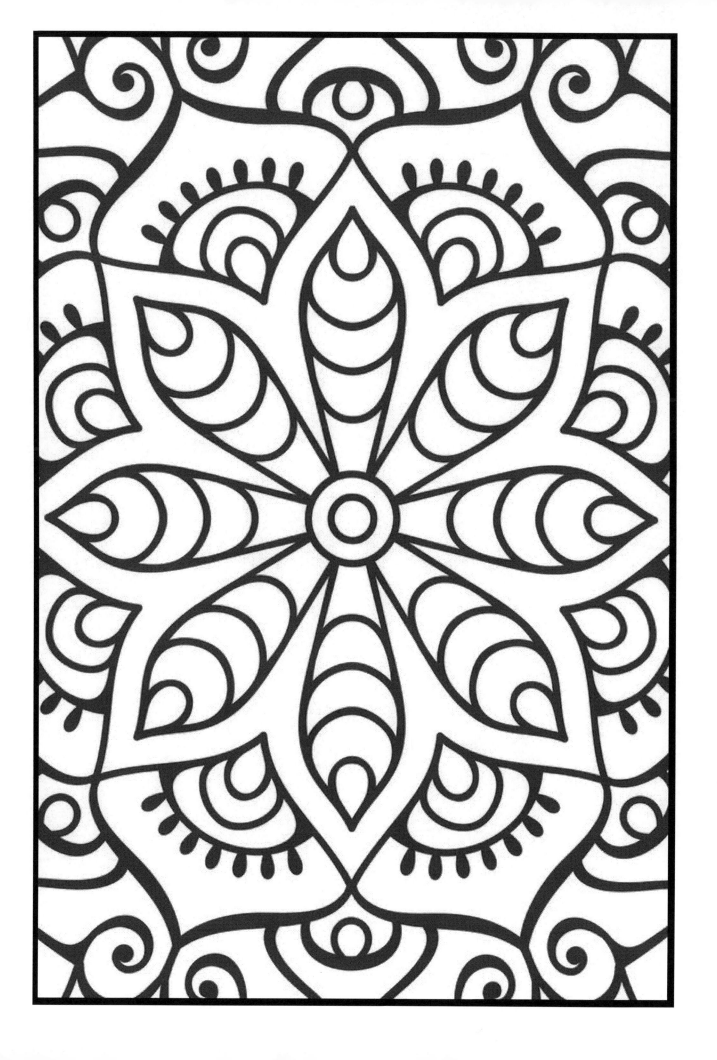

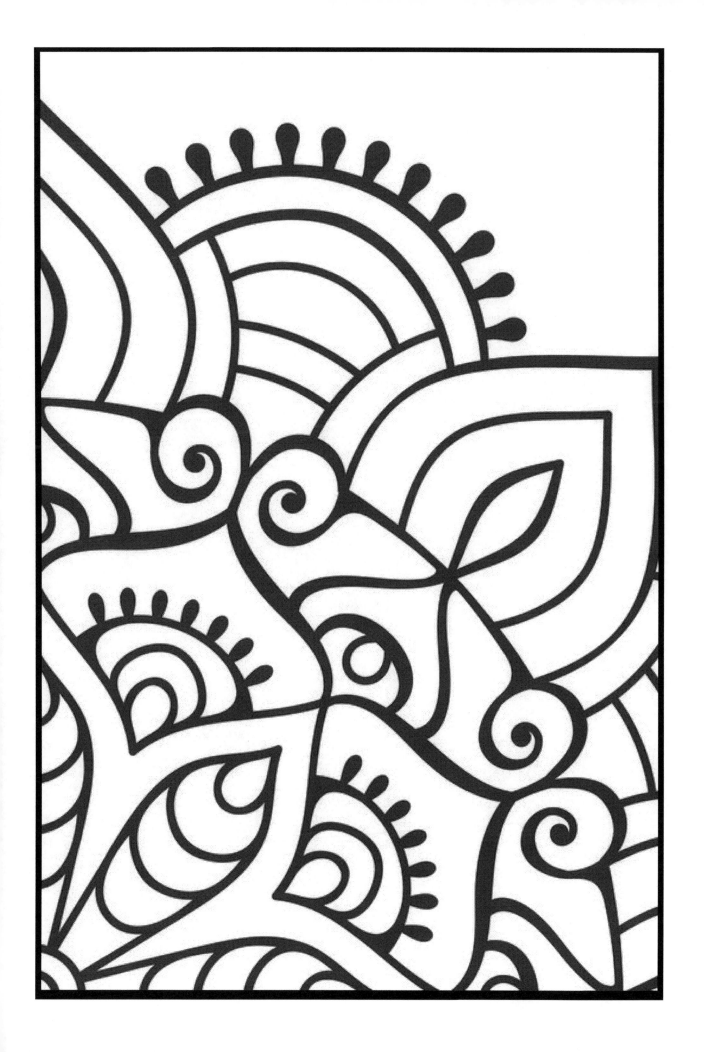

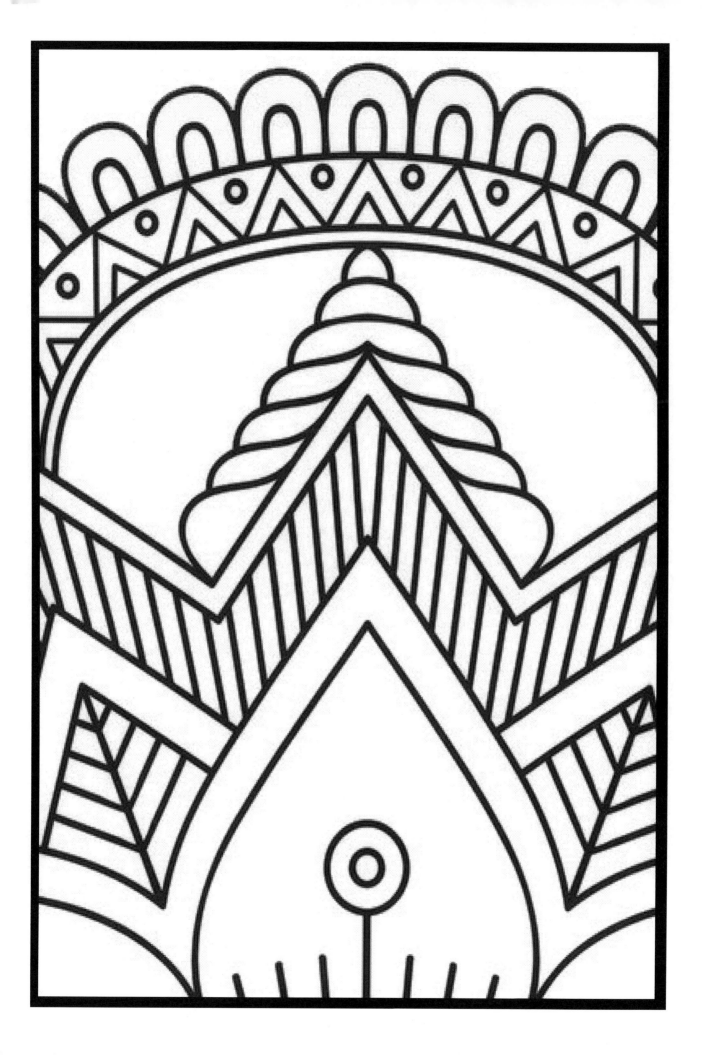

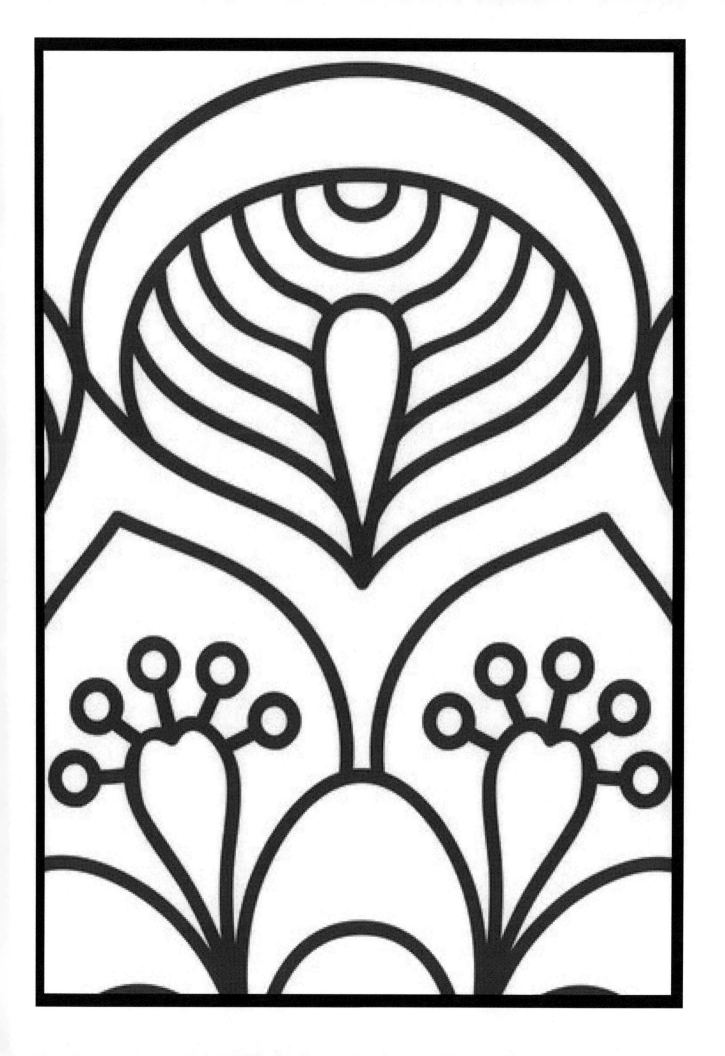

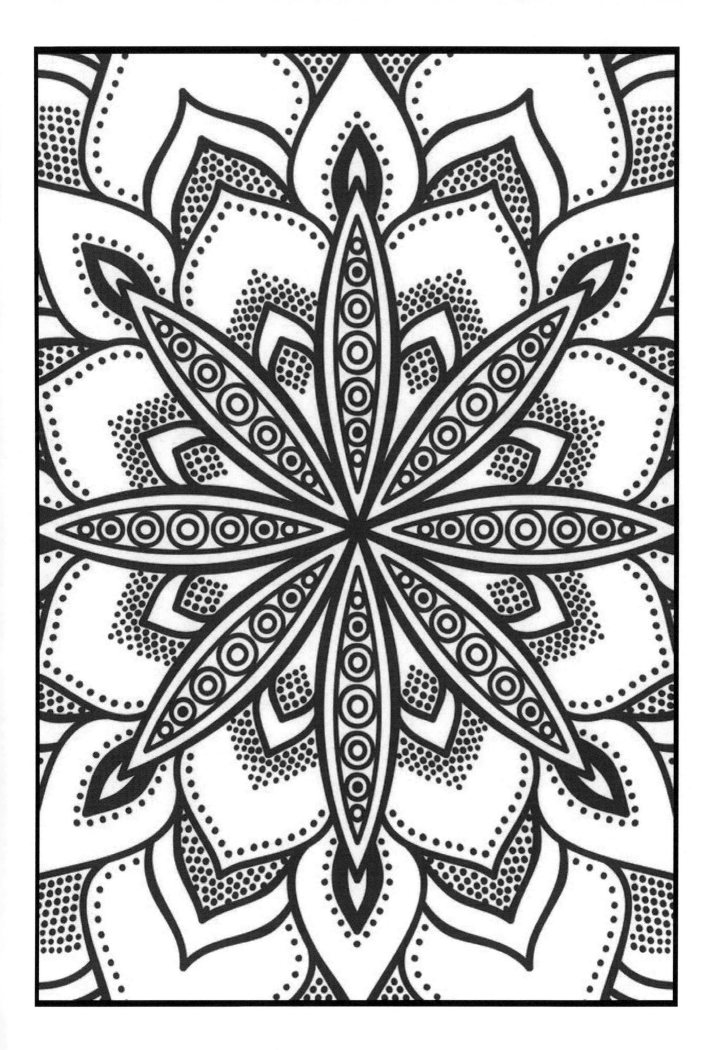

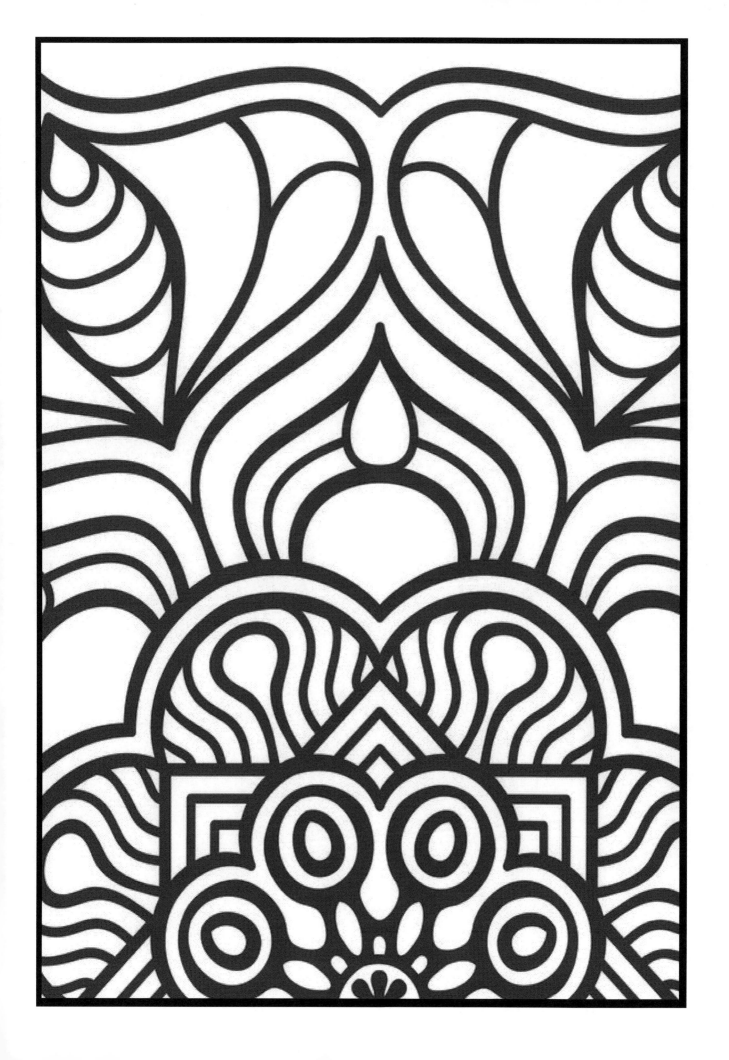

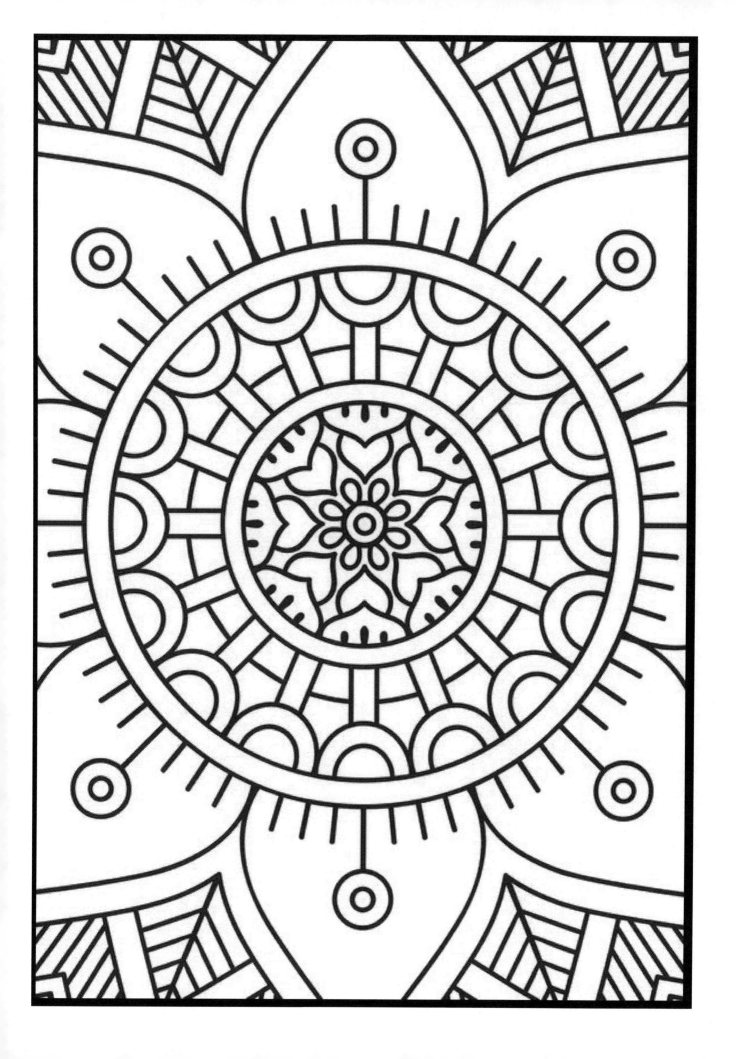

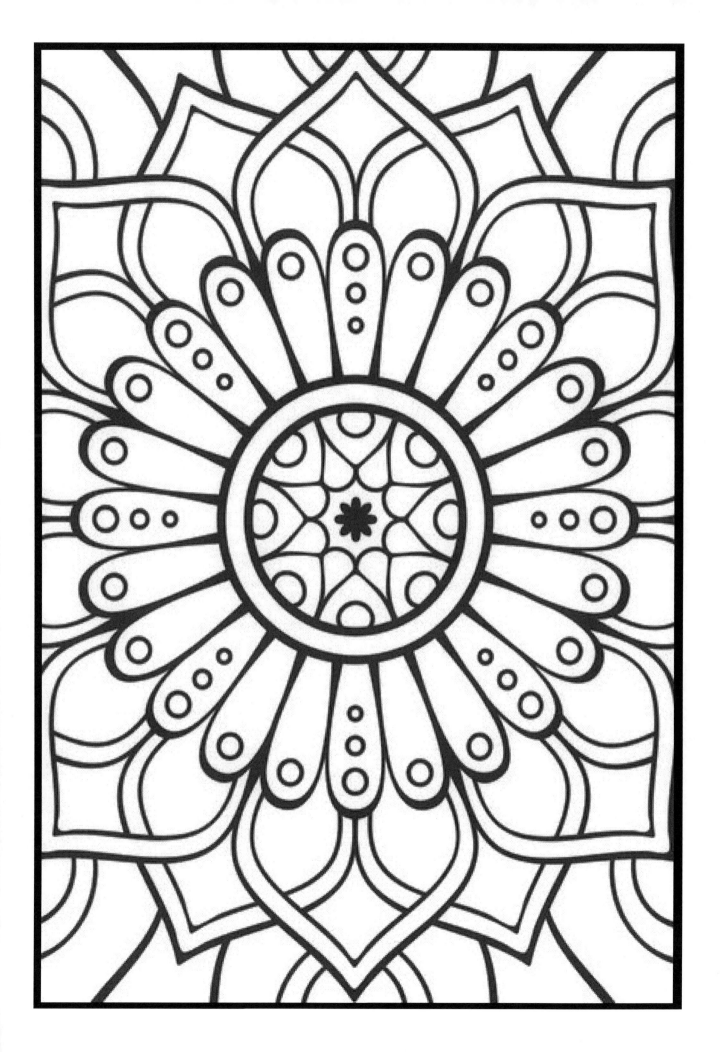

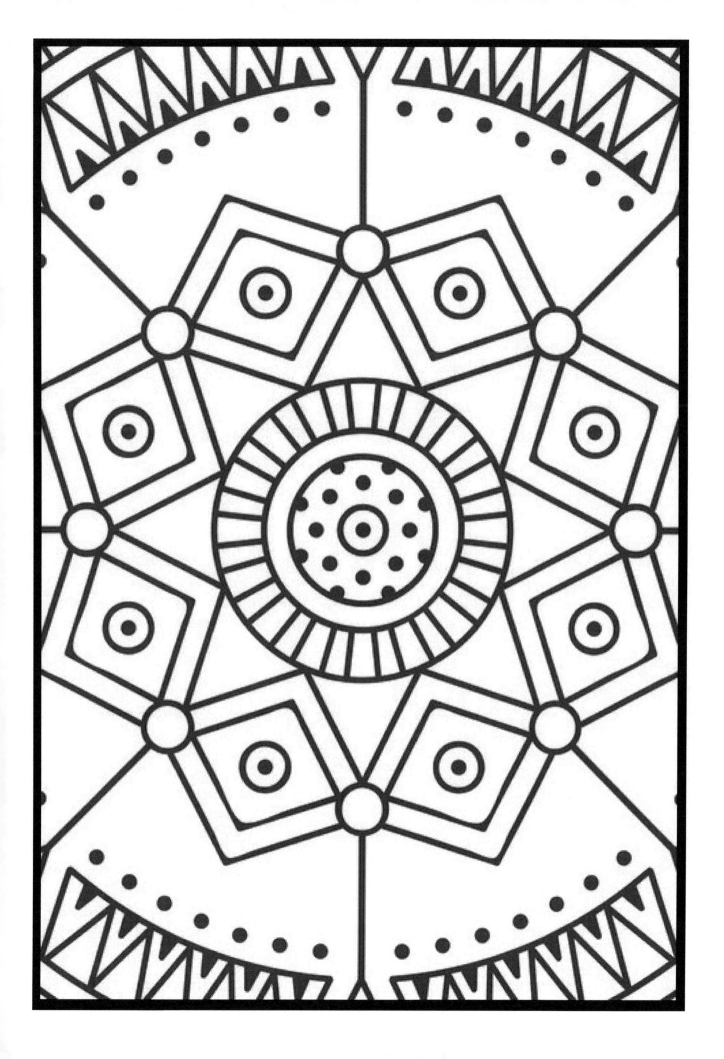

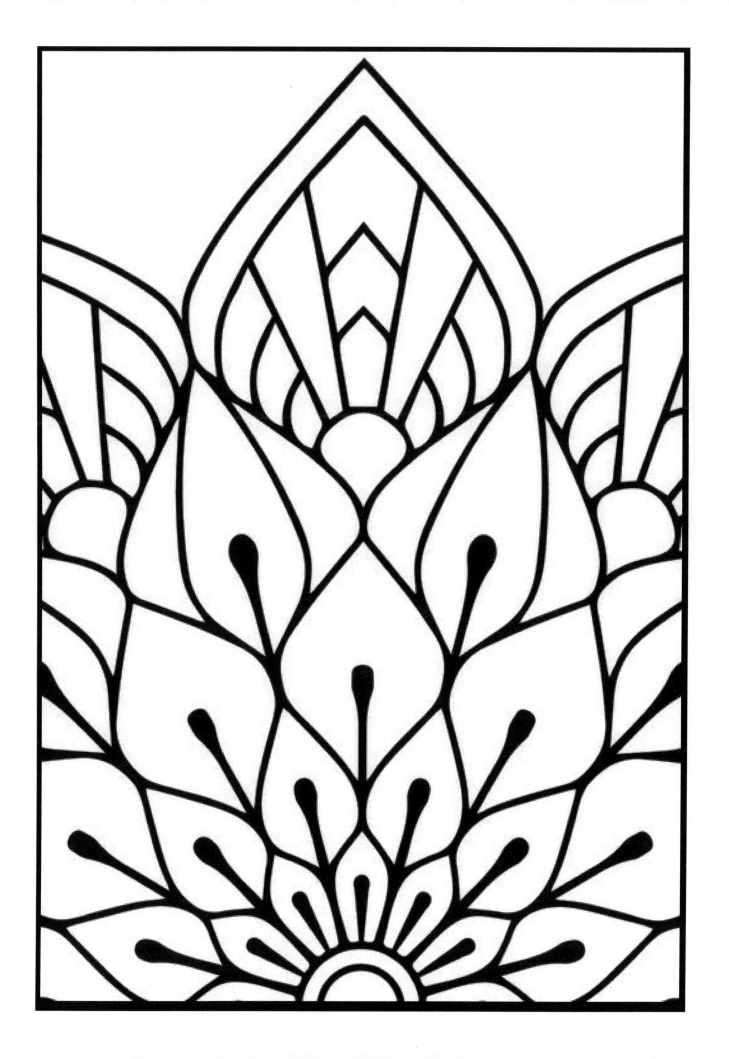

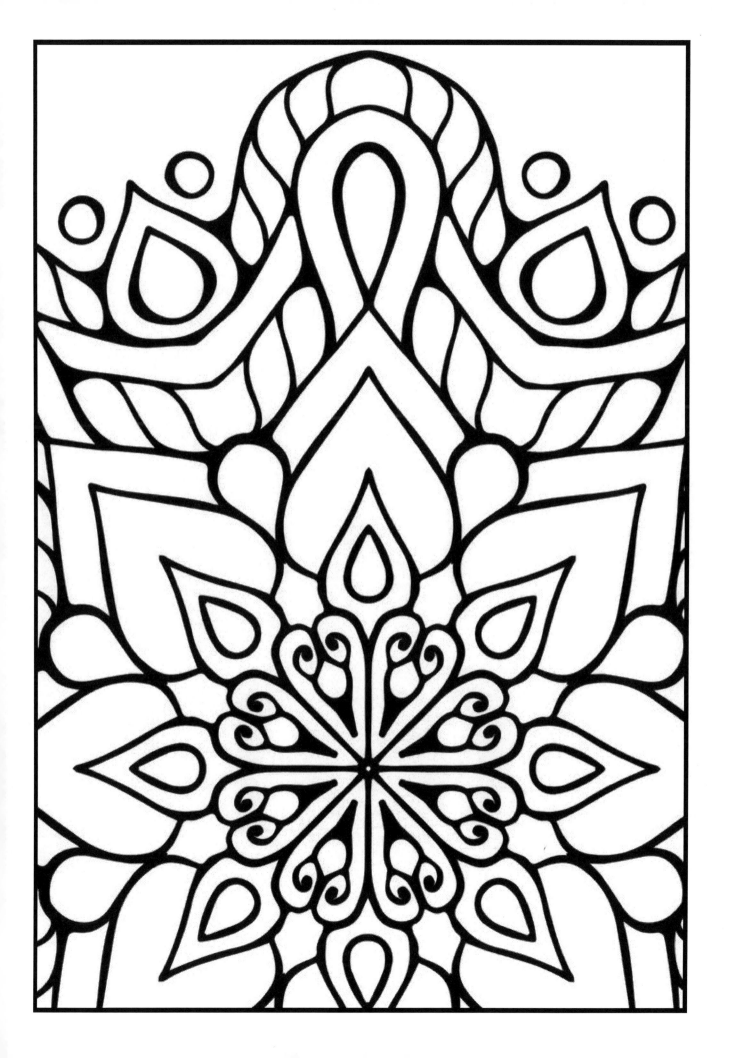

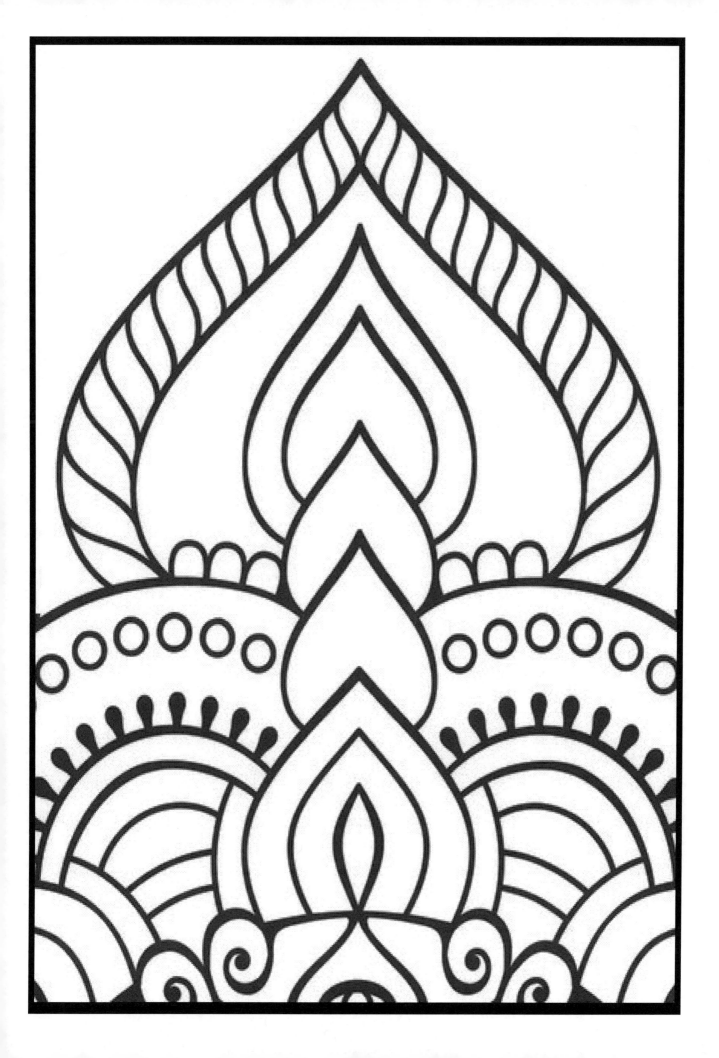

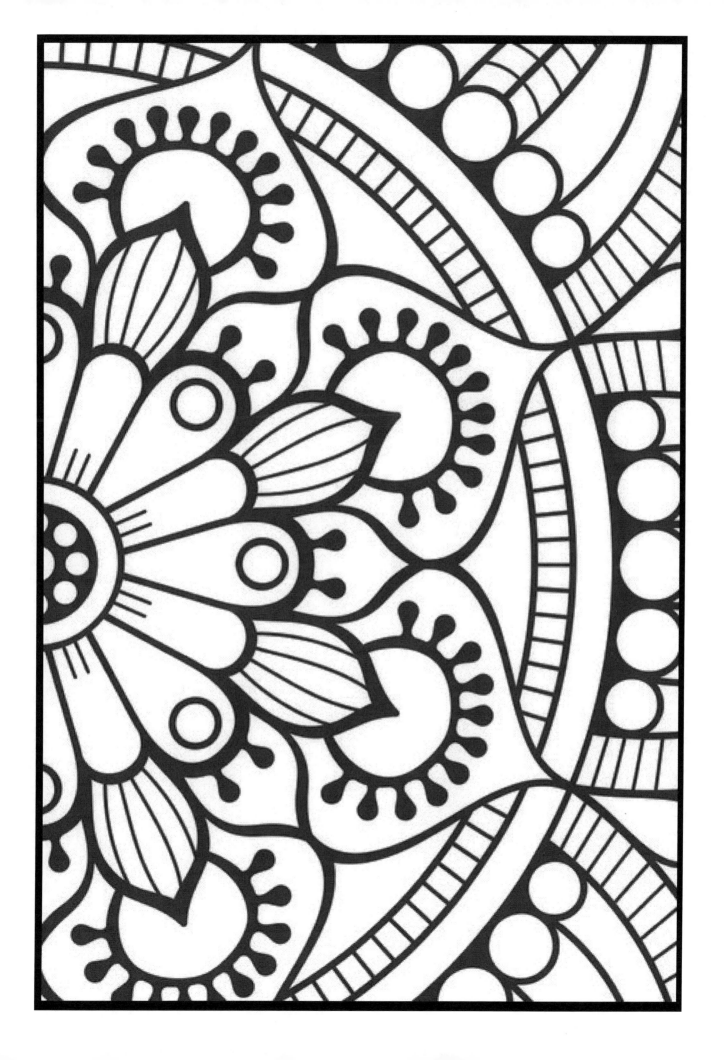

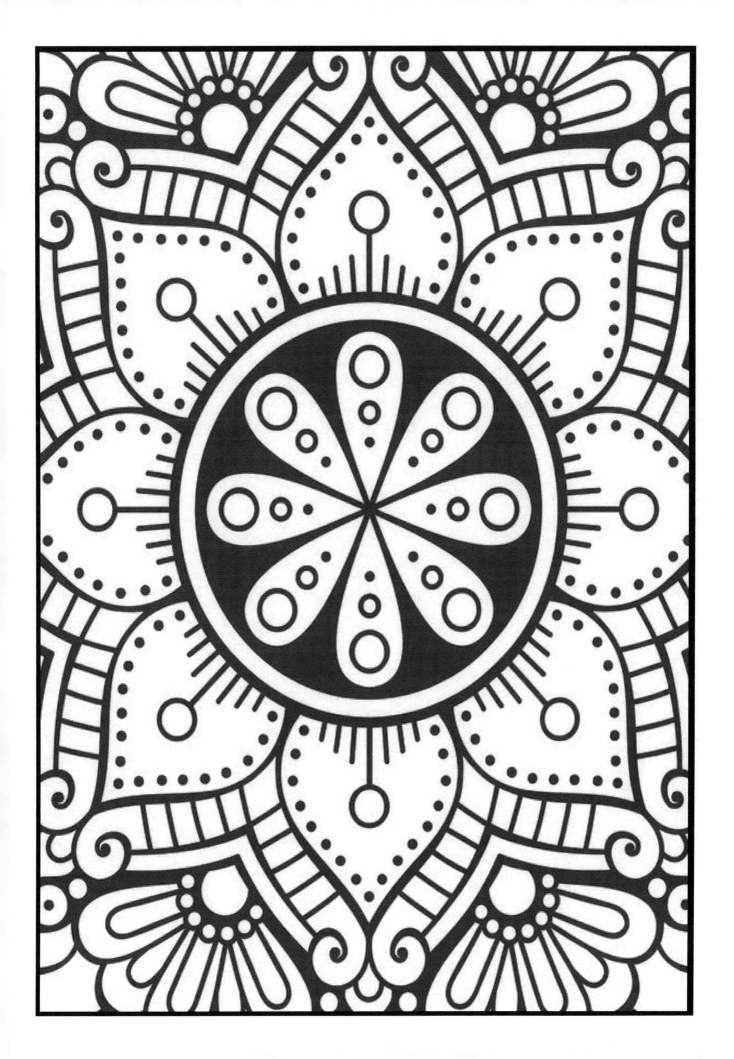

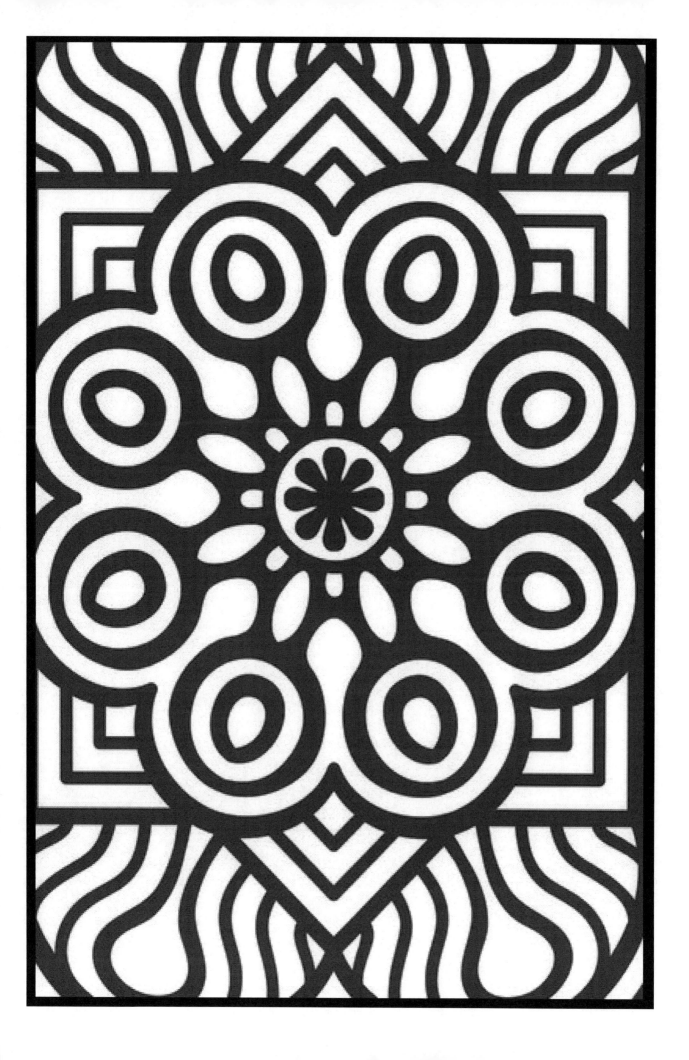

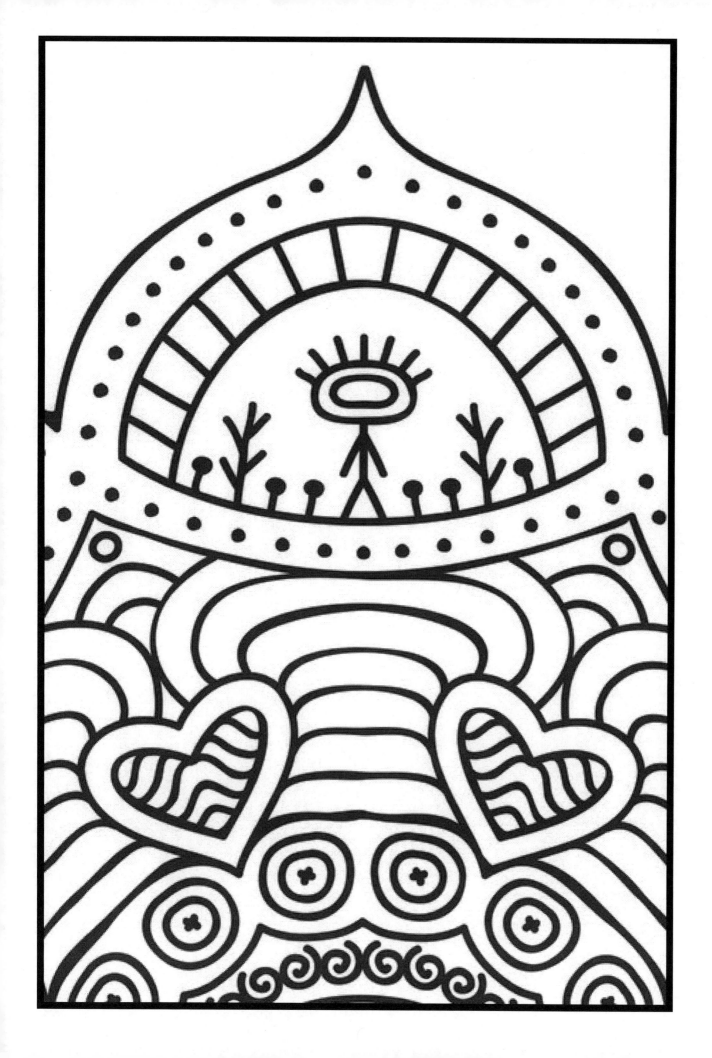

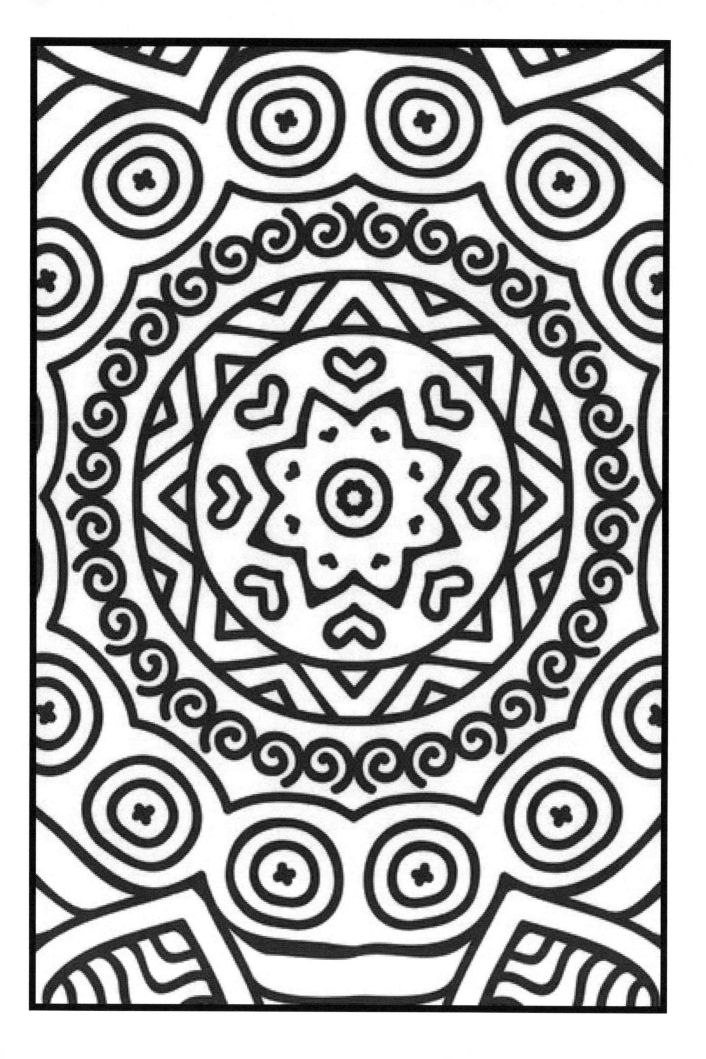

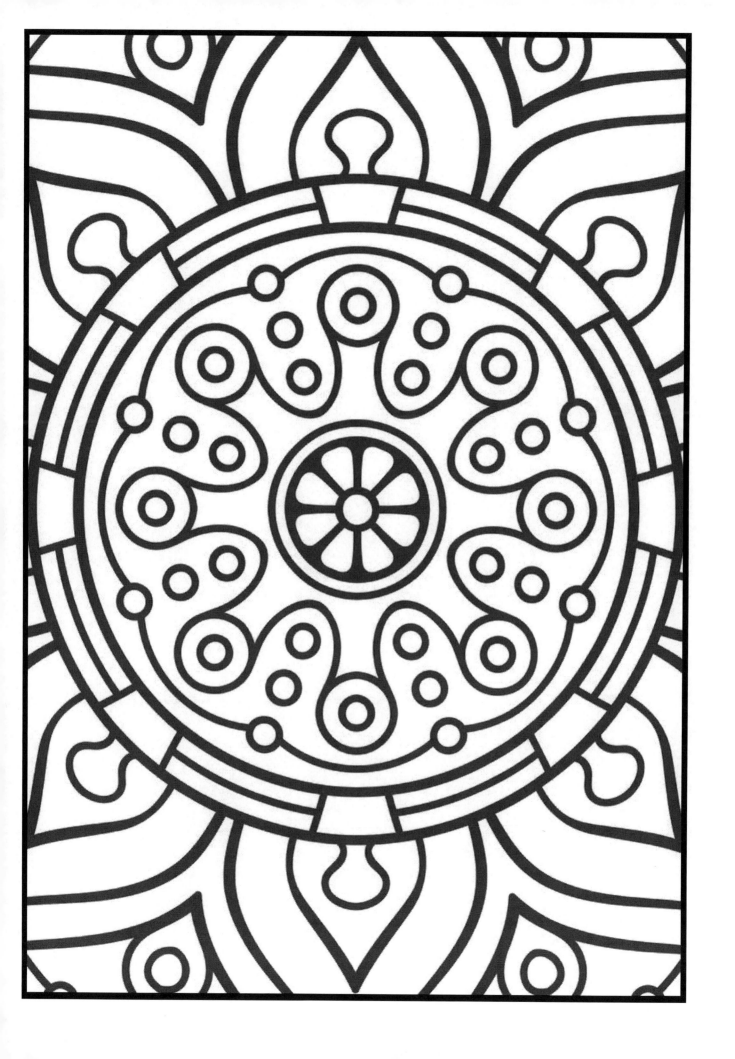

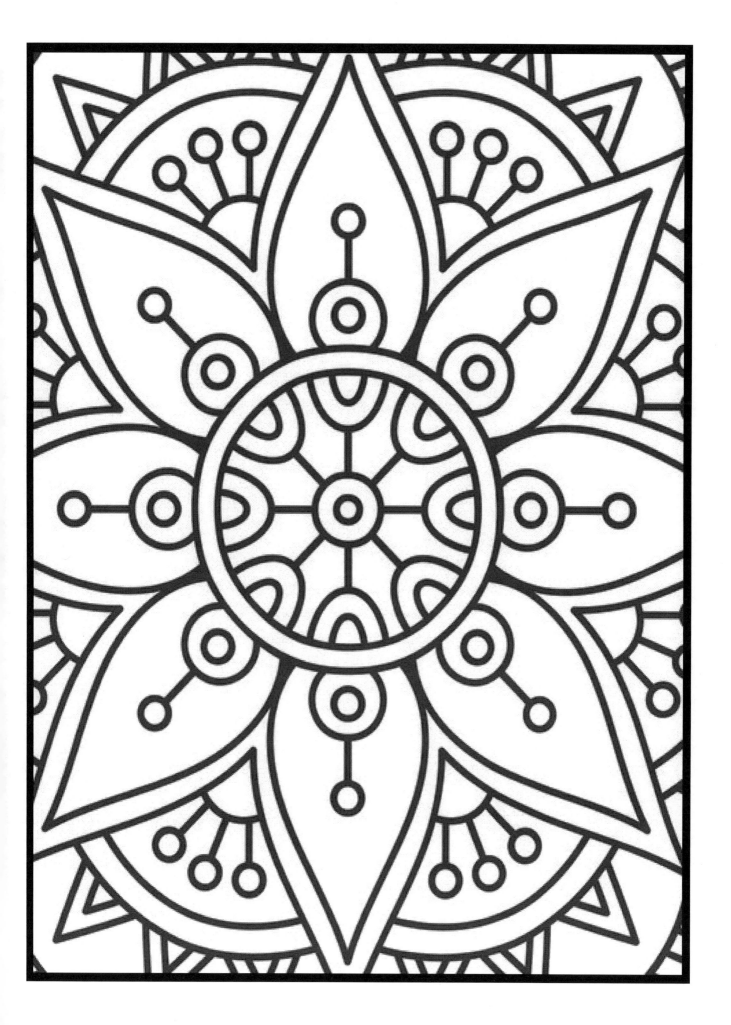

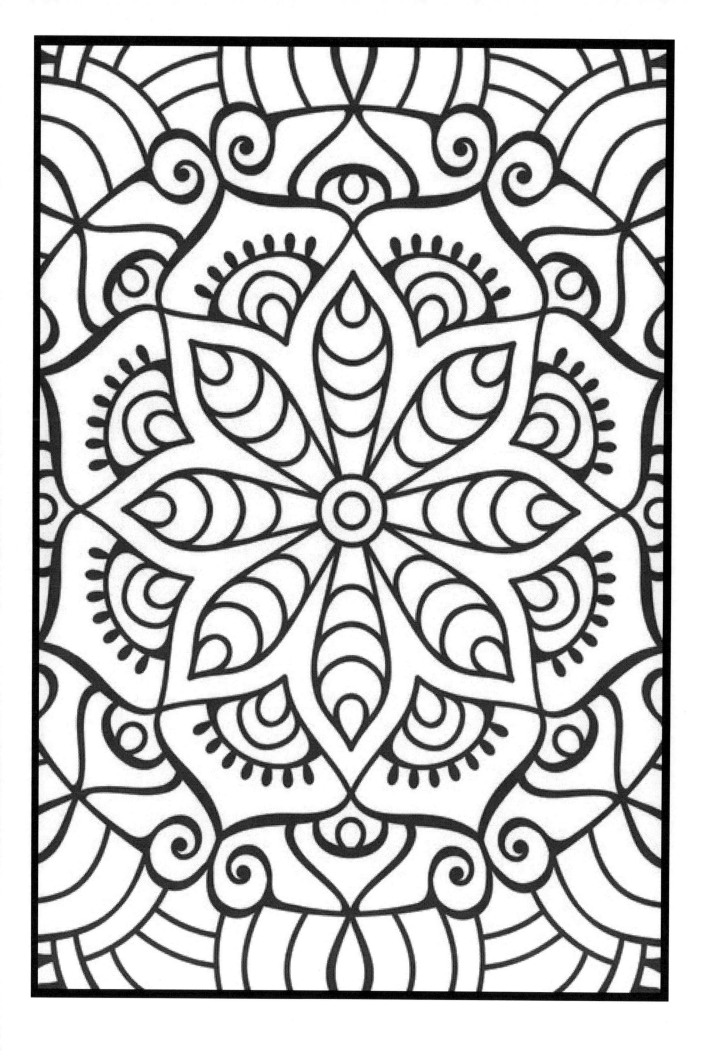

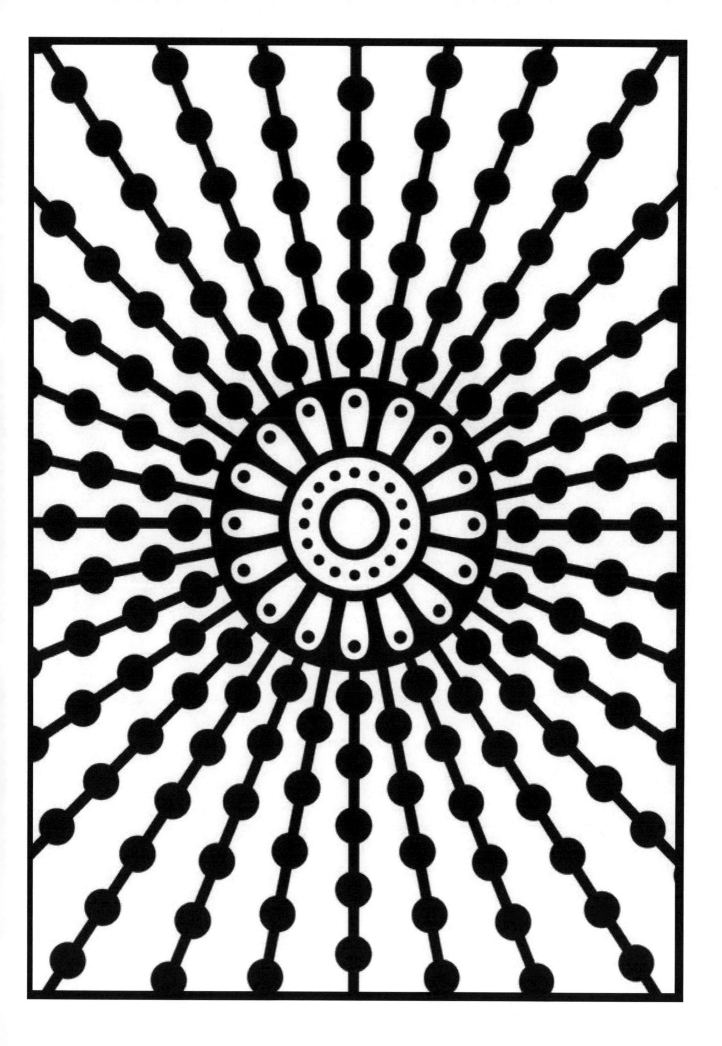

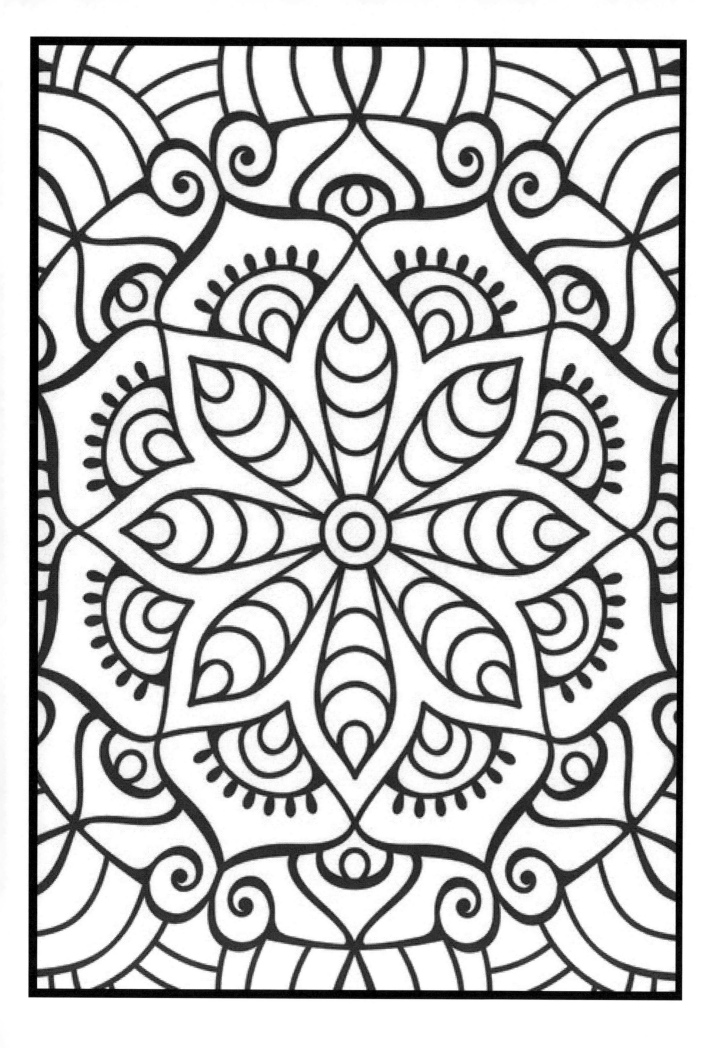

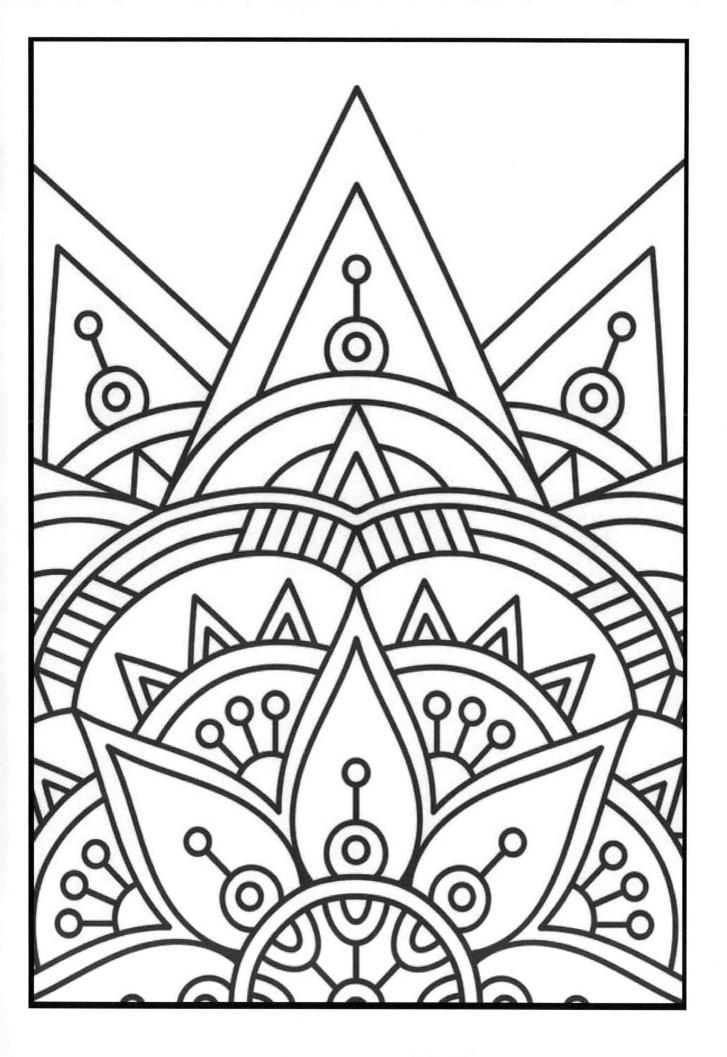

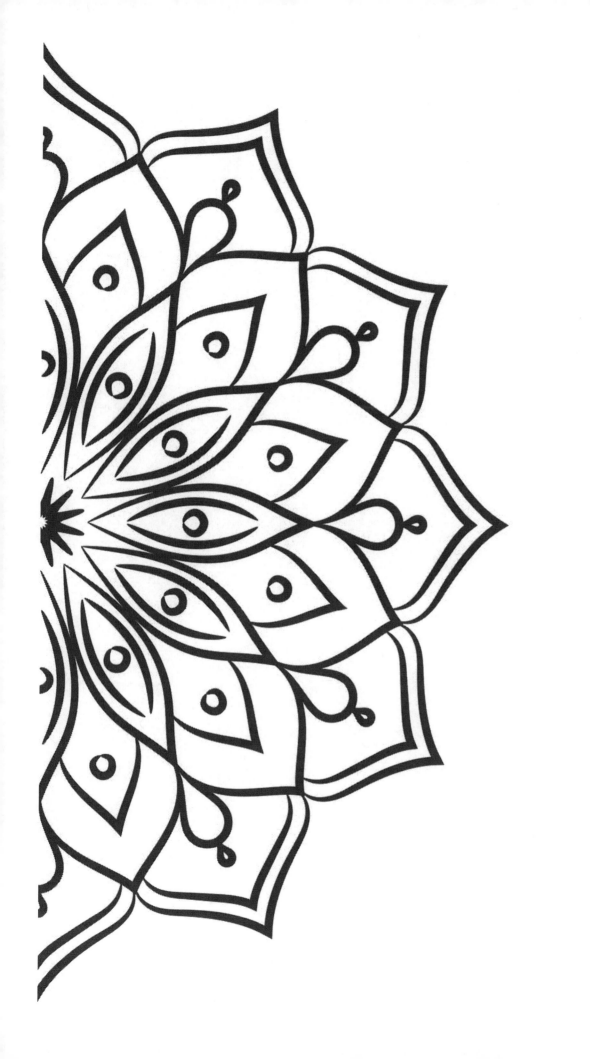

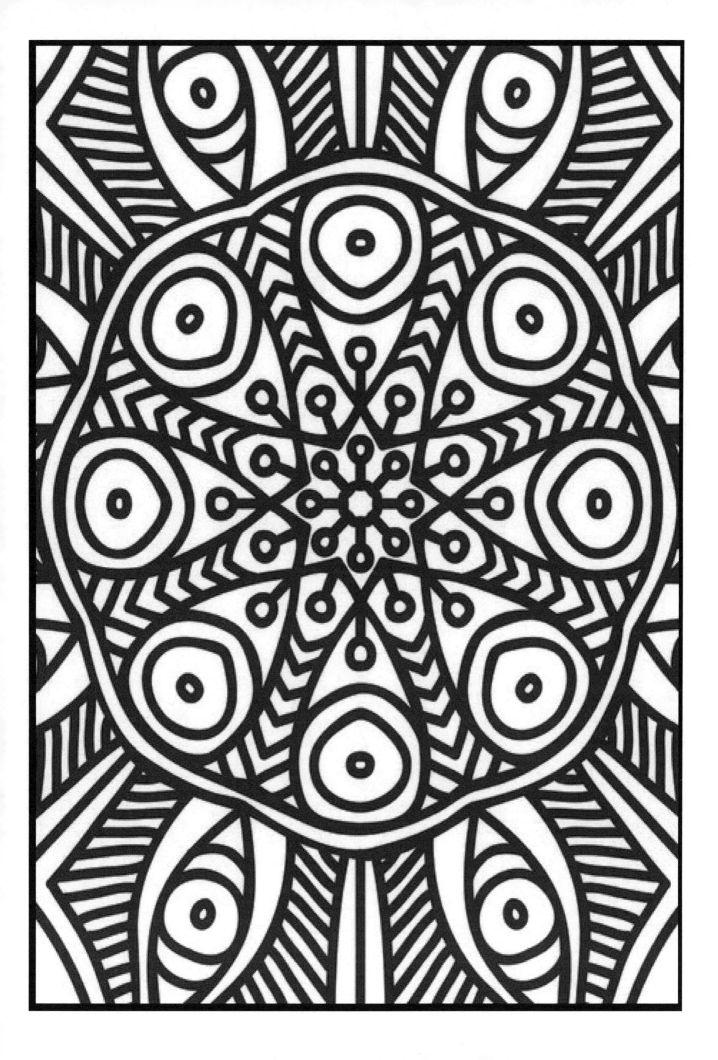

Thank you for coloring with us

Please review THIS book

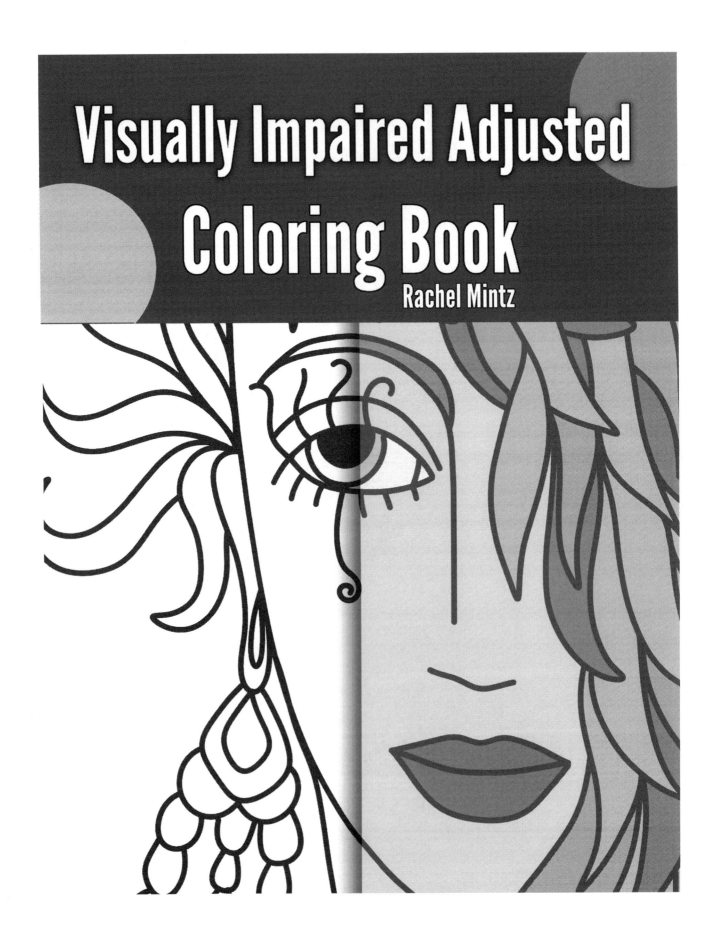

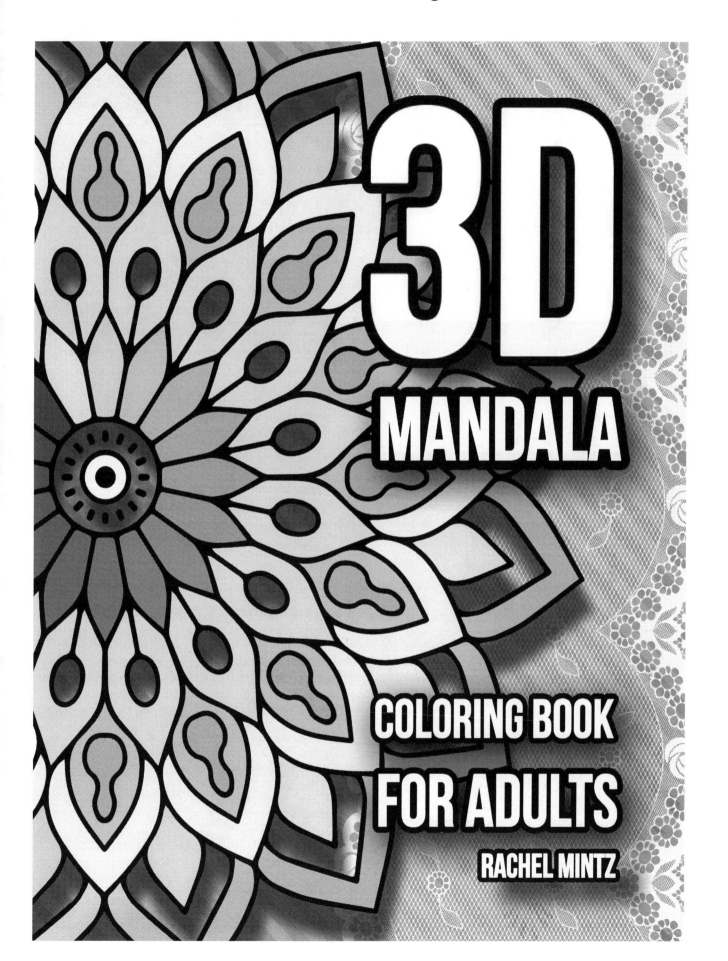

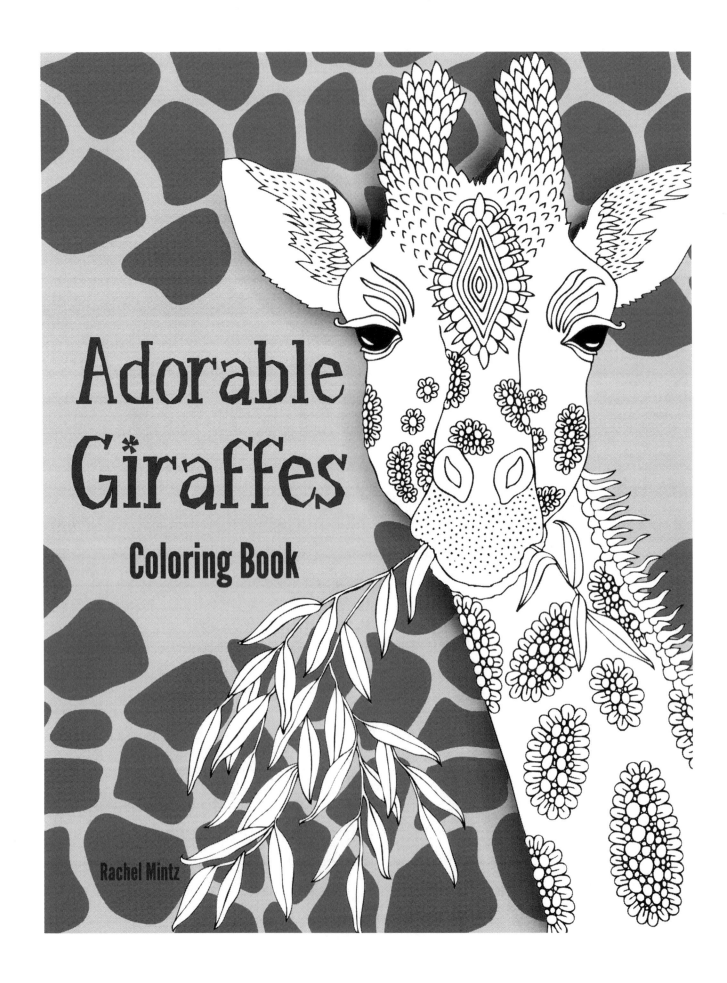

Adorable Giraffes

Coloring Book

Rachel Mintz

My Coffee Break

Coloring Book

Rachel Mintz

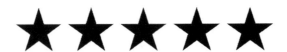

Thank you for coloring with us

We will be very thankful if you could take 60 seconds to review THIS book